The Keto Chaffle Easy Cookbook

Tasty and Delicious Recipes to Burn Fat

Kade Harrison

Table of Contents

Raspberry-Yogurt Chaffle Bowl

Preparation time:

10 minutes

Cooking time:

14 minutes

Servings: 2

Ingredients:

- 1 egg, beaten
- 1 tbsp almond flour
- ¼ cup finely grated mozzarella cheese
- ¼ tsp baking powder
- 1 cup Greek yogurt
- 1 cup fresh raspberries
- 2 tbsp almonds, chopped

Directions:

1. Preheat a waffle bowl maker and grease lightly with cooking spray.
2. Meanwhile, in a medium bowl, whisk all the ingredients except the yogurt, raspberries until smooth batter forms.
3. Open the iron, pour in half of the mixture, cover, and cook until crispy, 6 to 7 minutes.
4. Remove the chaffle bowl onto a plate and set aside.
5. Make the second chaffle bowl with the remaining batter.

6. To serve, divide the yogurt into the chaffle bowls and top with the raspberries and almonds.

Bacon-Cheddar Biscuit Chaffle

Preparation time:

10 minutes

Cooking time:

28 minutes

Servings: 4

Ingredients:

- 1 egg, beaten
- 2 tbsp almond flour
- 2 tbsp ground flaxseed
- 3 bacon slices, cooked and chopped
- ¼ cup heavy cream
- 1 ½ tbsp melted butter
- ½ cup finely grated Gruyere cheese
- ½ cup finely grated cheddar cheese
- ¼ tsp erythritol
- ½ tsp onion powder
- ½ tsp garlic salt
- ½ tbsp dried parsley
- ½ tbsp baking powder
- ¼ tsp baking soda

Directions:

1. Preheat the waffle iron.
2. Meanwhile, in a medium bowl, whisk all the ingredients until smooth batter forms.

3. Open the iron, pour a quarter of the mixture into the iron, close and cook until crispy, 6 to 7 minutes.
4. Remove the chaffle onto a plate and set aside.
5. Make three more Chaffles with the remaining batter.
6. Allow cooling and serve afterward.

Turnip Hash Brown Chaffles

Preparation time:

10 minutes

Cooking time:

42 minutes

Servings: 6

Ingredients:

- 1 large turnip, peeled and shredded
- ½ medium white onion, minced
- 2 garlic cloves, pressed
- 1 cup finely grated Gouda cheese
- 2 eggs, beaten
- Salt and freshly ground black pepper to taste

Directions:

1. Pour the turnips in a medium safe microwave bowl, sprinkle with 1 tbsp of water, and steam in the microwave until softened, 1 to 2 minutes.
2. Remove the bowl and mix in the remaining ingredients except for a quarter cup of the Gouda cheese.
3. Preheat the waffle iron.
4. Once heated, open and sprinkle some of the reserved cheese in the iron and top with 3 tablespoons of the mixture. Close the waffle iron and cook until crispy, 5 minutes.

5. Open the lid, flip the chaffle and cook further for 2 more minutes.
6. Remove the chaffle onto a plate and set aside.
7. Make five more chaffles with the remaining batter in the same proportion.
8. Allow cooling and serve afterward.

Everything Bagel Chaffles

Preparation time:

10 minutes

Cooking time:

28 minutes

Servings: 4

Ingredients:

- 1 egg, beaten
- ½ cup finely grated Parmesan cheese
- 1 tsp Everything Bagel seasoning

Directions:

1. Preheat the waffle iron.
2. In a medium bowl, mix all the ingredients.
3. Open the iron, pour in a quarter of the mixture, close, and cook until crispy, 6 to 7 minutes.
4. Remove the chaffle onto a plate and set aside.
5. Make three more chaffles, allow cooling, and enjoy after.

Blueberry Shortcake Chaffles

Preparation time:

10 minutes

Cooking time:

14 minutes

Servings: 2

Ingredients:

- 1 egg, beaten
- 1 tbsp cream cheese, softened
- ¼ cup finely grated mozzarella cheese
- 1/4 tsp baking powder
- 4 fresh blueberries
- 1 tsp blueberry extract

Directions:

1. Preheat the waffle iron.
2. In a medium bowl, mix all the ingredients.
3. Open the iron, pour in half of the batter, close, and cook until crispy, 6 to 7 minutes.
4. Remove the chaffle onto a plate and set aside.
5. Make the other chaffle with the remaining batter.

6. Allow cooling and enjoy after.

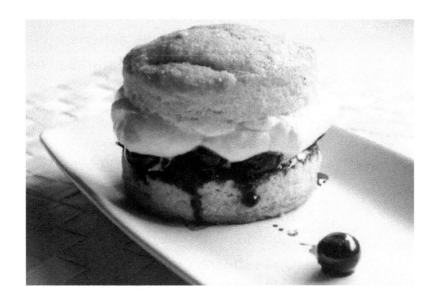

Raspberry-Pecan Chaffles

Preparation time:

10 minutes

Cooking time:

14 minutes

Servings: 2

Ingredients:

- 1 egg, beaten
- ½ cup finely grated mozzarella cheese
- 1 tbsp cream cheese, softened
- 1 tbsp sugar-free maple syrup
- ¼ tsp raspberry extract
- ¼ tsp vanilla extract
- 2 tbsp sugar-free caramel sauce for topping
- 3 tbsp chopped pecans for topping

Directions:

1. Preheat the waffle iron.
2. In a medium bowl, mix all the ingredients.
3. Open the iron, pour in half of the batter, close, and cook until crispy, 6 to 7 minutes.
4. Remove the chaffle onto a plate and set aside.
5. Make another chaffle with the remaining batter.

6. To serve: drizzle the caramel sauce on the chaffles and top with the pecans.

Breakfast Spinach Ricotta Chaffles

Preparation time:

10 minutes

Cooking time:

28 minutes

Servings: 4

Ingredients:

- 4 oz frozen spinach, thawed, squeezed dry
- 1 cup ricotta cheese
- 2 eggs, beaten
- ½ tsp garlic powder
- ¼ cup finely grated Pecorino Romano cheese
- ½ cup finely grated mozzarella cheese
- Salt and freshly ground black pepper to taste

Directions:

1. Preheat the waffle iron.
2. In a medium bowl, mix all the ingredients.
3. Open the iron, lightly grease with cooking spray and spoon in a quarter of the mixture.
4. Close the iron and cook until brown and crispy, 7 minutes.
5. Remove the chaffle onto a plate and set aside.

6. Make three more chaffles with the remaining mixture.
7. Allow cooling and serve afterward.

Scrambled Egg Stuffed Chaffles

Preparation time:

15 minutes

Cooking time:

28 minutes

Servings: 4

Ingredients:

- For the chaffles:
- 1 cup finely grated cheddar cheese
- 2 eggs, beaten
- For the egg stuffing:
- 1 tbsp olive oil
- 4 large eggs
- 1 small green bell pepper, deseeded and chopped
- 1 small red bell pepper, deseeded and chopped
- Salt and freshly ground black pepper to taste
- 2 tbsp grated Parmesan cheese

Directions:

1. For the chaffles:
2. Preheat the waffle iron.In a medium bowl, mix the cheddar cheese and egg.

3. Open the iron, pour in a quarter of the mixture, close, and cook until crispy, 6 to 7 minutes.
4. Plate and make three more chaffles using the remaining mixture.
5. For the egg stuffing:
6. Meanwhile, heat the olive oil in a medium skillet over medium heat on a stovetop.
7. In a medium bowl, beat the eggs with the bell peppers, salt, black pepper, and Parmesan cheese.
8. Pour the mixture into the skillet and scramble until set to your likeness, 2 minutes.
9. Between two chaffles, spoon half of the scrambled eggs and repeat with the second set of chaffles.
10.   Serve afterward.

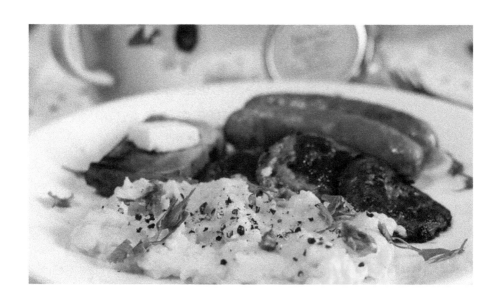

Mixed Berry-Vanilla Chaffles

Preparation time:

10 minutes

Cooking time:

28 minutes

Servings: 4

Ingredients:

- 1 egg, beaten
- ½ cup finely grated mozzarella cheese
- 1 tbsp cream cheese, softened
- 1 tbsp sugar-free maple syrup
- 2 strawberries, sliced
- 2 raspberries, slices
- ¼ tsp blackberry extract
- ¼ tsp vanilla extract
- ½ cup plain yogurt for serving

Directions:

1. Preheat the waffle iron.
2. In a medium bowl, mix all the ingredients except the yogurt.
3. Open the iron, lightly grease with cooking spray and pour in a quarter of the mixture.
4. Close the iron and cook until golden brown and crispy, 7 minutes.
5. Remove the chaffle onto a plate and set aside.

6. Make three more chaffles with the remaining mixture.
7. To serve: top with the yogurt and enjoy.

Ham and Cheddar Chaffles

Preparation time:

15 minutes

Cooking time:

28 minutes

Servings: 4

Ingredients:

- 1 cup finely shredded parsnips, steamed
- 8 oz ham, diced
- 2 eggs, beaten
- 1 ½ cups finely grated cheddar cheese
- ½ tsp garlic powder
- 2 tbsp chopped fresh parsley leaves
- ¼ tsp smoked paprika
- ½ tsp dried thyme
- Salt and freshly ground black pepper to taste

Directions:

1. Preheat the waffle iron.
2. In a medium bowl, mix all the ingredients.

3. Open the iron, lightly grease with cooking spray and pour in a quarter of the mixture.
4. Close the iron and cook until crispy, 7 minutes.
5. Remove the chaffle onto a plate and set aside.
6. Make three more chaffles using the remaining mixture.
7. Serve afterward.

Savory Gruyere and Chives Chaffles

Preparation time:

15 minutes

Cooking time:

14 minutes

Servings: 2

Ingredients:

- 2 eggs, beaten
- 1 cup finely grated Gruyere cheese
- 2 tbsp finely grated cheddar cheese
- 1/8 tsp freshly ground black pepper
- 3 tbsp minced fresh chives + more for garnishing
- 2 sunshine fried eggs for topping

Directions:

1. Preheat the waffle iron.
2. In a medium bowl, mix the eggs, cheeses, black pepper, and chives.
3. Open the iron and pour in half of the mixture.
4. Close the iron and cook until brown and crispy, 7 minutes.
5. Remove the chaffle onto a plate and set aside.
6. Make another chaffle using the remaining mixture.

7. Top each chaffle with one fried egg each, garnish with the chives and serve.

Chicken Quesadilla Chaffle

Preparation time:

10 minutes

Cooking time:

14 minutes

Servings: 2

Ingredients:

- 1 egg, beaten
- ¼ tsp taco seasoning
- 1/3 cup finely grated cheddar cheese
- 1/3 cup cooked chopped chicken

Directions:

1. Preheat the waffle iron.
2. In a medium bowl, mix the eggs, taco seasoning, and cheddar cheese. Add the chicken and combine well.
3. Open the iron, lightly grease with cooking spray and pour in half of the mixture.
4. Close the iron and cook until brown and crispy, 7 minutes.
5. Remove the chaffle onto a plate and set aside.
6. Make another chaffle using the remaining mixture.

7. Serve afterward.

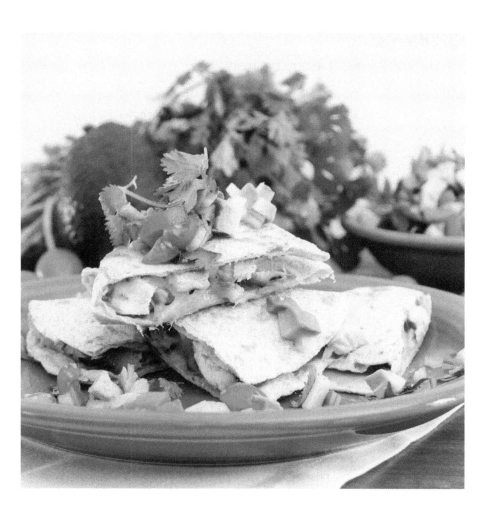

Hot Chocolate Breakfast Chaffle

Preparation time:

10 minutes

Cooking time:

14 minutes

Servings: 2

Ingredients:

- 1 egg, beaten
- 2 tbsp almond flour
- 1 tbsp unsweetened cocoa powder
- 2 tbsp cream cheese, softened
- ¼ cup finely grated Monterey Jack cheese
- 2 tbsp sugar-free maple syrup
- 1 tsp vanilla extract

Directions:

1. Preheat the waffle iron.
2. In a medium bowl, mix all the ingredients.
3. Open the iron, lightly grease with cooking spray and pour in half of the mixture.
4. Close the iron and cook until crispy, 7 minutes.
5. Remove the chaffle onto a plate and set aside.
6. Pour the remaining batter in the iron and make the second chaffle.

7. Allow cooling and serve afterward.

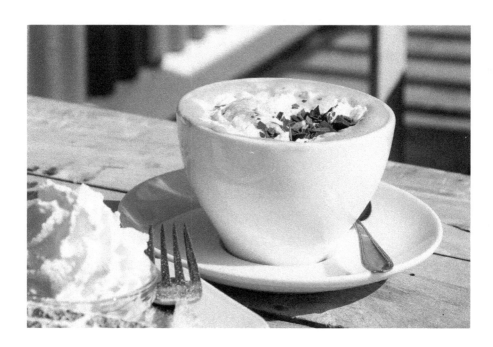

Chicken Cauli Chaffle

Preparation time:

27 minutes

Cooking time:

12 minutes

Servings: 2

Ingredients:

- Chicken: 3-4 pieces or ½ cup when done
- Garlic: 2 cloves (finely grated)
- Egg: 2
- Salt: As per your taste
- Green onion: 1 stalk
- Soy Sauce: 1 tablespoon
- Cauliflower Rice: 1 cup
- Mozzarella cheese: 1 cup
- Black pepper: ¼ teaspoon or as per your taste
- White pepper: ¼ teaspoon or as per your taste

Directions:

1. Melt some butter in an oven and set aside, then cook the chicken in a skillet using salt and a cup of water to boil. With the lid closed, cook for 18 minutes.

2. Once done, put off the heat and shred the chicken into pieces, then discard all bones.

3. Using another mixing bowl prepare a mix containing peppers (white and black), soy sauce, cauliflower rice, grated garlic, beaten egg with the shredded chicken pieces.

4. Mix evenly. Preheat and grease the waffle maker.

5. Pour 1/8 cup of mozzarella into the waffle maker with the mixture on the cheese, add another cup (1/8) of mozzarella on the chaffle. With a closed lid, heat the waffle for 5 minutes to a crunch and then remove the chaffle.

6. Repeat for the remaining chaffles mixture to make more batter.

7. Serve by garnishing the chaffle with chopped green onions and enjoy.

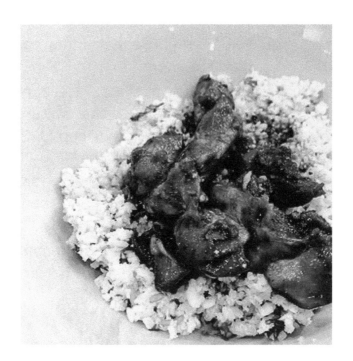

Garlic Chicken Chaffle

Preparation time:

27 minutes

Cooking time:

12 minutes

Servings: 2

Ingredients:

- Chicken: 3-4 pieces
- Garlic: 1 clove
- Egg: 1
- Salt
- Lemon juice: ½ tablespoon
- Kewpie mayo: 2 tablespoon
- Mozzarella cheese: ½ cup

Directions:

1. Cook the chicken in a skillet using salt and a cup of water to boil.
2. With the lid closed, cook for 18 minutes.
3. Once done, put off the heat and shred the chicken into pieces, then discard all bones.
4. Using another mixing bowl prepare a mix containing 1/8 cup of cheese, Kewpie mayo, lemon juice and grated garlic.
5. Mix evenly. Preheat and grease the waffle maker.
6. Arrange chaffles on a baking tray with the chicken, then sprinkle cheese on the chaffles.

7. With a closed lid, heat the waffle for 5 minutes until cheese melts and then remove the chaffle.
8. Repeat for the remaining chaffles mixture to make more batter.
9. Serve and warm.

Buffalo Chicken Chaffle

Preparation time:

12 minutes

Cooking time:

6 minutes

Servings: 2

Ingredients:

- Egg: 2
- Buffalo sauce: 4 tablespoons (can be as desired)
- Chicken: 1 cup
- Cheddar Cheese: 1 cup
- Softened cream cheese: ¼ cup
- Butter: 1 teaspoon

Directions:

1. Melt some butter in a pan with shredded chicken added into it.
2. Add tablespoons of buffalo sauce into the heated mix. Using a mixing bowl, prepare a mixture containing eggs with whipped cream cheese, cheddar cheese and cooked chicken, then mix evenly.
3. Preheat and grease a waffle maker.
4. Sprinkle some cheddar cheese at the base of the waffle maker, then the mixture spread evenly on the waffle maker with a bit of cheese.
5. Heat to a crispy form for 5 minutes and repeat the process for the remaining batter.

6. Serve the dish with some buffalo sauce to enjoy.

Chicken Mozzarella Chaffle

Preparation time:

12 minutes

Cooking time:

6 minutes

Servings: 2

Ingredients:

- Chicken: 1 cup
- Mozzarella cheese: 1 cup and 4 tablespoons
- Basil: ½ teaspoon
- Butter: 1 teaspoon
- Egg: 2
- Tomato sauce: 6 tablespoons
- Garlic: ½ tablespoon

Directions:

1. Melt some butter in a pan with shredded chicken added into it and stir for few minutes.
2. Add basil with garlic and set aside.
3. Using a mixing bowl, prepare a mixture containing eggs with cooked chicken and mozzarella cheese, then mix evenly.
4. Preheat and grease a waffle maker.
5. Spread the mixture on the base of the mini-waffle maker evenly, then heat for 5 minutes to a crispy form.
6. Repeat the process for the remaining batter.

7. On a baking tray, arrange the chaffles with tomato sauce and grated cheese to garnish the top.
8. Heat the oven at 399F to melt cheese then serve best hot.

Chicken Bbq Chaffle

Preparation time:

32 minutes

Cooking time:

11 minutes

Servings: 2

Ingredients:

- Chicken: 1/2 cup
- BBQ sauce: 1 tablespoon (sugar-free)
- Egg: 1
- Almond flour: 2 tablespoon
- Cheddar cheese: ½ cup
- Butter: 1 tablespoon

Directions:

1. Melt some butter in a pan with shredded chicken added into it and stir for 11 minutes.
2. Using a mixing bowl, prepare a mixture containing all ingredients with the cooked chicken, then mix evenly.
3. Preheat and grease a waffle maker.
4. Spread the mixture on the base of the waffle maker evenly, and then heat for 7 minutes to a crispy form.
5. Repeat the process for the remaining batter.
6. Serve best hot.

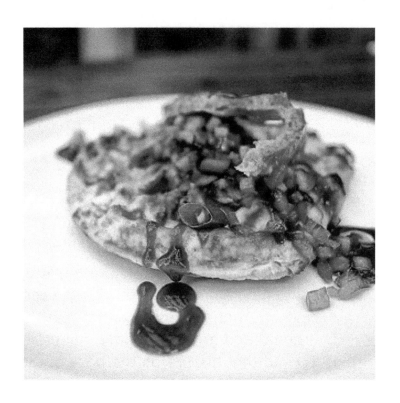

Chicken Spinach Chaffle

Preparation time:

41 minutes

Cooking time:

11 minutes

Servings: 2

Ingredients:

- Spinach: ½ cup
- Pepper: As per your taste
- Basil: 1 teaspoon
- Chicken: ½ cup boneless
- Shredded mozzarella: half cup
- Garlic powder: 1 tablespoon
- Salt: As per your taste
- Egg: 1
- Onion powder: 1 tablespoon

Directions:

1. Heat the chicken in water to boil, then shred it into pieces and keep aside. Heat the spinach for 9 minutes to strain.
2. Using a mixing bowl, prepare a mixture containing all ingredients with the cooked chicken, then mix evenly.
3. Preheat and grease a waffle maker.
4. Spread the mixture on the base of the waffle maker evenly, and then heat for 7 minutes to a crispy form.
5. Repeat the process for the remaining batter.

6. Serve best crispy with your desired keto
   sauce.

Chicken Parmesan Chaffle

Preparation time:

30 minutes

Cooking time:

5 minutes

Ingredients:

- 1/2 Cup Canned Chicken Breast Or Leftover Shredded Chicken
- 1/4 Cup Cheddar Cheese
- 1/8 Cup Parmesan Cheese
- 1 Egg
- 1 Teaspoon Italian Seasoning
- 1/8 Teaspoon Garlic Powder
- 1 Teaspoon Cream Cheese, Room Temperature
- Topping Ingredients
- 2 Slices Of Provolone Cheese
- 1 Tablespoon Sugar-Free Pizza Sauce

Directions:

1. Preheat the mini waffle maker.
2. In a medium-size bowl, add all the ingredients and mix until it's fully incorporated.
3. Add a teaspoon of shredded cheese to the waffle iron for 30 seconds before adding the mixture.
4. This will create the best crust and make it easier to take this heavy

chaffle out of the waffle maker when it's done.

5. Pour half of the mixture in the mini waffle maker and cook it for a minimum of 4 to 5 minutes.

6. Repeat the above steps to cook the second Chicken Parmesan Chaffle.

7. Top with a sugar-free pizza sauce and one slice of provolone cheese.

Corndog Chaffle

Preparation time:

45 minutes

Cooking time:

5 minutes

Ingredients:

- 2 Eggs
- 1 Cup Mexican Cheese Blend
- 1 Tablespoon Almond Flour
- 1/2 Teaspoon Cornbread Extract
- 1/4 Teaspoon Salt
- Hot Dogs With Hot Dog Sticks
- Optional: For Extra Added Spice Be Sure To Add Diced Jalapenos To This Recipe!

Directions:

1. Preheat corndog waffle maker.
2. In a small bowl, whip the eggs.
3. Add the remaining ingredients, except for the hotdogs
4. Spray the corndog waffle maker with non-stick cooking spray.
5. Fill the corndog waffle maker with the batter halfway filled. (if you want a crispy corndog, add a small amount of cheese 30 seconds before adding the batter)
6. Place a stick in the hot dog.

7. Place the hot dog in the batter and slightly press down.

8. Spread a small amount of batter on top of the hot dog, just enough to fill it.

9. Makes about 4 to 5 chaffle corndogs

10. Cook the corndog chaffles for about 4 minutes or until golden brown.

11. When done, they will easily remove from the corndog waffle maker with a pair of tongs.

12. Serve with mustard, mayo, or sugar-free ketchup!

Burger Bun Chaffle

Preparation time:

3 minutes

Cooking time:

5 minutes

Ingredients:

- 1 Large Egg, Beaten
- 1/2 Cup Shredded Mozzarella
- 1 Tb Almond Flour
- 1/4 Tsp Baking Powder
- 1 Teaspoon Sesame Seeds
- 1 Pinch Of Onion Powder

Directions:

1. Combine all ingredients
2. Pour half into a mini waffle maker (or split between two)
3. Cook for 5 minutes or until you no longer see steam coming from the waffle maker.
4. Remove to a wire rack and allow to cool.

Halloumi Cheese Chaffle

Preparation time:

5 minutes

Cooking time:

5 minutes

Ingredients:

- 3 Ounces Halloumi Cheese
- 2 Tablespoons Pasta Sauce Optional

Directions:

1. Cut Halloumi cheese into 1/2 inch thick slices.
2. Place cheese in the UNHEATED waffle maker.
3. Turn waffle maker on.
4. Let it cook for about 3-6 minutes or until golden brown and to your liking.
5. Let it cool for some time on a rack.
6. Add Low Carb marinara or pasta sauce.
7. Serve immediately. Enjoy!

Keto Sausage Ball Chaffle Recipe

Preparation Time:

10 minutes

Cooking Time:

5 minutes

Serving: 3

Ingredients:

- 1 Pound Bulk Italian
- 1 Cup Sharp Cheddar
- Sausage
- Cheese
- 1 Cup Almond Flour
- 1/4 Cup Parmesan
- 2 Tsp Baking Powder
- Cheese
- 1 Egg

Directions:

1. Preheat the smaller than normal Chaffle producer.
2. Consolidate all ingredient in an enormous blending bowl and blend well utilizing your hands.
3. Spot a paper plate under Chaffle creator to get any spillage.
4. Scoop 3 T of blend onto warmed Chaffle creator.
5. Cook for at least 3 minutes.
6. Flip over and cook 2

7. Additional minutes for even firmness.

Pumpkin Cake Chaffle

Preparation Time:

10 minutes

Cooking Time:

10 minutes

Serving: 4

Ingredients:

- 1 Egg
- Frosting
- 1/2 Cup Mozzarella
- Ingredients:
- Cheese
- 2 Tbs Cream Cheese
- 1/2 Tsp Pumpkin Pie
- 2 Tbs Monkfruit
- Spice
- Confectioners Blend
- 1 Tbs Pumpkin
- 1/2 Tsp Clear Vanilla Extract

Directions:

1. Preheat the little Chaffle producer.
2. In a little bowl, whip the egg.
3. Include the cheddar, pumpkin pie flavor, and the pumpkin.
4. Include 1/2 of the blend to the little Chaffle producer and cook it for at any rate 3 to 4 minutes until it's brilliant darker.

5. While the chaffle is cooking, include the entirety of the cream cheddar icing ingredients in a bowl and blend it until it's smooth and rich.
6. On the off chance that you need a rich taste to this icing, you can likewise include a tbs of genuine margarine that has been relaxed at room
7. temperature.
8. Add the cream cheddar icing to the hot chaffle and serve it right away.

Keto Lemon Chaffle Recipe

Preparation Time:

10 minutes

Cooking Time:

10 minutes

Serving: 4

Ingredients:

- Chaffle Cake:
- 20 Drops Cake
- 2- Oz Cream Cheese
- Batter Extract
- 2 Eggs
- Chaffle Frosting:
- 2 Tsp Butter
- 1/2 Cup Heavy
- 2 Tbs Coconut Flour
- Whipping Cream
- 1 Tsp Monkfruit
- 1 Tbs Monkfruit
- 1 Tsp Baking Powder
- 1/4 Tsp Lemon
- 1/2 Tsp Lemon Extract

Directions:

1. Preheat the smaller than normal Chaffle producer 67
2. Include the entirety of the elements for the chaffle cake in a blender and blend it until the hitter is decent and

smooth. This should just take a few minutes.

3. Utilize a dessert scoop and fill the Chaffle iron with one full scoop of hitter. This size of the frozen yogurt scoop is around 3 tsp and fits superbly in the smaller than usual Chaffle producer.

4. While the chaffles are cooking, start making the icing.

5. In a medium-size bowl, include the chaffle icing ingredients.

6. Blend the ingredients until the icing is thick with tops.

7. All the chaffles to totally cool before icing the cake

8. Discretionary: Add lemon strip for additional flavor!

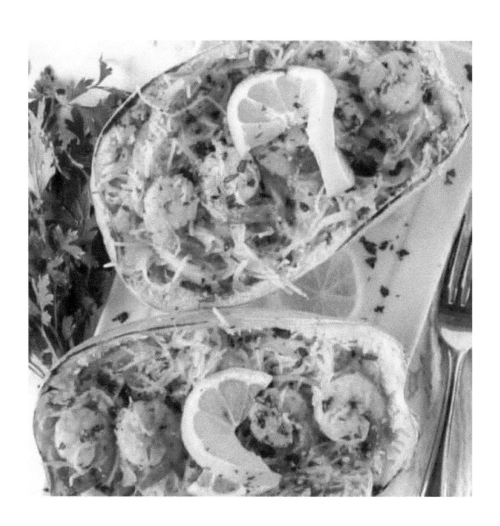

Cinnamon Roll Chaffles

Preparation Time:

5 minutes

Cooking Time:

15 minutes

Serving: 2

Ingredients:

- 2- large eggs
- 1/2 tsp. kosher salt
- 2- tbsp. almond
- 1/2- tsp. baking
- flour
- soda
- tsp. pure vanilla
- c. shredded
- extract
- mozzarella
- tbsp. granulated
- Cooking spray:
- swerve
- oz. cream cheese
- 1/2- tsp. cinnamon
- tbsp. heavy cream

Directions:

1. Preheat Chaffle iron to high. In an enormous bowl, beat eggs.
2. Mix in almond flour, vanilla, 1 tsp 69

3. swerve, cinnamon, salt, and preparing pop. Toss in mozzarella.
4. Oil Chaffle iron with cooking shower, at that point
5. Pour portion of the hitter into the
6. Chaffle iron and cook until light brilliant, around 3 minutes.
7. Rehash with the outstanding hitter.
8. In a medium microwave-safe bowl, join cream cheddar, substantial cream, and staying 1 tsp swerve. Microwave, whisking like clockwork, until softened and drizzly
9. Top Chaffles with strawberries and sprinkle with cream cheddar blend and maple syrup.

Keto Cheese Chaffle Recipe

Preparation Time:

10 minutes

Cooking Time:

8 minutes

Serving: 2

Ingredients:

- 1 large egg
- 1/2 c. shredded cheese
- Pinch of salt
- Seasoning

Directions:

1. Preheat the scaled-down Chaffle producer, in a bowl, whisk the egg until beaten.
2. Shred the cheddar
3. Include the cheddar, salt, and flavoring to the egg, at that point blend well.
4. Scoop half of the blend on the Chaffle producer spread uniformly.
5. Cook 3-4 minutes, until done exactly as you would prefer, pull it off and let cool.
6. Include the remainder of the hitter and cook the second Chaffle.
7. Enjoy

Maple Pumpkin Keto Chaffle Recipe

Preparation Time:

5 minutes

Cooking Time:

16 minutes

Servings: 2

Ingredients:

- 2 eggs
- 2 tsp Lakanto
- 3/4 tsp baking
- Sugar-Free Maple
- powder
- Syrup
- 2 tsp pumpkin
- 1 tsp coconut flour
- puree
- 1/2 cup mozzarella
- 3/4 tsp pumpkin
- cheese
- pie spice
- 1/2 tsp vanilla
- 4 tsp heavy
- Pinch of salt
- whipping cream

Directions:

1. Turn on Chaffle or chaffle creator. I utilize the Dash Mini, Chaffle Maker.
2. In a little bowl, join all ingredients.

63

3. Spread the scramble smaller than expected Chaffle creator with 1/4 of the hitter and cook for 3-4
4. minutes.
5. Rehash 3 additional occasions until you have made 4 Maple Syrup
6. Pumpkin Keto Chaffles

Mini Keto Pizza Recipe

Preparation Time:

5 minutes

Cooking Time:

10 minutes

Servings: 2 Mini Keto Pizzas

Ingredients:

- 1/2 cup Shredded
- 1/4 tsp garlic
- Mozzarella cheese
- powder
- 1 tsp almond flour
- 1/4 tsp basil
- 1/2 tsp baking
- 2 tsp low carb pasta
- powder
- sauce
- 1 eggs
- 2 tsp mozzarella
- cheese

Directions:

1. While the Chaffle creator is warming up, in a bowl blend mozzarella cheddar, heating powder, garlic, premise, egg and almond flour.

2. Pour 1/2 the blend into your smaller than normal Chaffle producer.

3. Cook for 3-5 minutes until your pizza Chaffle is totally cooked.

4. In the event that you check it and the Chaffle adheres to the Chaffle producer let it cook for one more moment or two.

5. Next put the rest of the pizza outside layer blend into the Chaffle producer and cook it.

6. When both pizza outsides are cooked, place them on the heating sheet of your toaster stove.

7. Put 1 tsp of low carb pasta sauce over every pizza outside layer.

8. Sprinkle 1 tsp of shredded mozzarella cheddar over everyone.

9. Heat at 350 degrees in the toaster broiler for about 5 minutes, just until the cheddar is softened 76

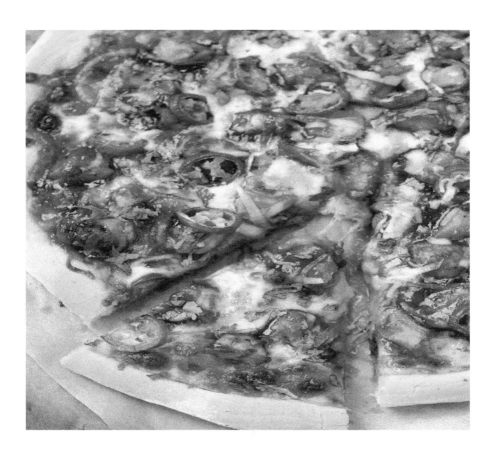

Perfect Pumpkin Spice Chaffles

Preparation Time:

15 minutes

Cooking Time:

5 minutes

Serving: 8

Ingredients:

- 4 large eggs
- pint buttermilk
- 2 1/4 tsp baking
- 1 cup canned solid-
- powder
- pack pumpkin
- 2 tsp ground
- 6 tsp unsalted
- cinnamon
- butter
- 1 tsp baking soda
- 2 1/2 cups all-
- 1 tsp ground ginger
- purpose flour
- 1/2 tsp salt
- 1/3 cup packed light
- 1/4 tsp ground
- brown sugar
- cloves

Directions:

1. Preheat a Chaffle iron
2. Beat egg whites in a glass or metallic bowl until delicate pinnacles shape. Lift your mixer or whisk immediately up: the egg whites will form delicate hills in place of a pointy pinnacle.
3. Beat egg yolks, buttermilk, pumpkin, and spread together with a velocity in a massive bowl until smooth; consist of flour, darker sugar, heating powder, cinnamon, making ready pop, ginger, salt, and cloves.
4. Mix the mixture with the whisk simply till you have a easy participant.
5. Overlay the egg whites into the participant just until consolidated.
6. Get geared up cooking surfaces of your Chaffle iron with cooking bathe.

7. Spoon round 2/3 cup participant into the readied iron and cook dinner until caramelized, four to 5 minutes.

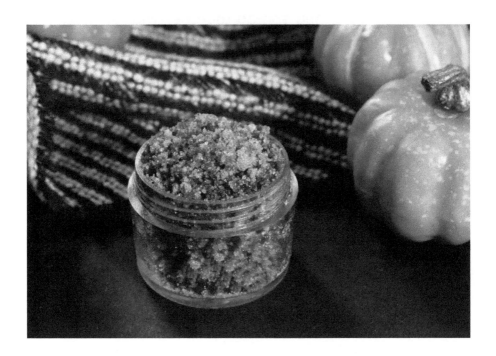

Banana Chaffles

Preparation Time:

10 minutes

Cooking Time:

30 minutes

Serving: 4

Ingredients

- 1 1/4 Cups All-
- 1 pinch ground
- purpose flour
- nutmeg
- 3 tsp baking powder
- 1 cup milk
- 1/2 tsp salt
- 1 egg
- 2 ripe bananas

Directions:

1. Preheat Chaffle iron. In a huge blending bowl, filter together flour, heating powder, salt, and nutmeg.
2. Mix in milk and eggs until the blend is smooth.
3. Splash preheated Chaffle iron with non-stick cooking shower. Pour two tsp of the Chaffle hitter onto the hot Chaffle iron.
4. Spot two cuts of banana over the hitter and afterward spoon another

two tsp of the batter over the banana.

5. Cook until brilliant dark colored.
6. Serve hot.

Gingerbread Chaffles With Hot Chocolate Sauce

Preparation Time:

25 minutes

Cooking Time:

25 minutes

Serving: 6

Ingredients:

- cup light
- ½- tsp ground
- molasses
- cinnamon
- ½- cup butter
- ½- tsp salt
- 1 ½- tsp baking
- cups boiling
- soda
- water
- ½- cup milk
- cup white sugar
- egg
- tsp cornstarch
- cups all-purpose
- ½- cup
- flour
- unsweetened cocoa
- 1 ½- tsp ground

- powder
- ginger
- tsp salt
- tsp vanilla
- tsp butter
- extract

Directions:

1. Remove from warmth and let cool somewhat. Mix in heating pop, milk, and egg.
2. In an enormous bowl, filter together flour, ginger, cinnamon, and salt.
3. Make a well in the middle and pour in the molasses blend.
4. Splash preheated Chaffle iron with non-stick cooking shower.
5. Pour blend into the hot Chaffle iron.
6. Cook until brilliant darker. Serve hot with chocolate sauce. To make chocolate sauce: In a pot, join water, 1 cup sugar, cornstarch, cocoa powder, and 1 tsp salt.
7. Cook over medium warmth, blending continually until blend reaches boiling point.
8. Remove from warmth and include vanilla and 2
9. Tsp spread; mix until smooth.

Kate's Light Fluffy Buttermilk And Chocolate Chip Chaffles

Preparation Time:

15 minutes

Cooking Time:

20 minutes,

Serving: 10

Ingredients

- 1 ½- cups all-
- ¼- cup heavy
- purpose flour
- cream
- tsp powdered
- egg yolks
- buttermilk
- ¼- cup butter
- 1 ¼- tsp baking
- egg whites
- powder
- cup miniature
- ½- tsp baking soda
- semisweet chocolate
- cup milk
- chips

Directions:

1. In an enormous bowl, blend the flour, powdered buttermilk, heating powder, and preparing pop.
2. In 83 a different bowl, whip the cream utilizing an electric blender; mix in milk, egg yolks, and dissolved margarine.
3. Mix the milk blend into the dry ingredients until smooth. In a spotless glass or metal bowl, whip egg whites to solid pinnacles.
4. Overlay the egg whites and chocolate chips into the batter utilizing an elastic spatula or wooden spoon.
5. Preheat a Chaffle iron, and coat with cooking shower.
6. Spoon batter onto the hot iron, and cook until there is never again steam turning out and the Chaffles are light dark-colored.

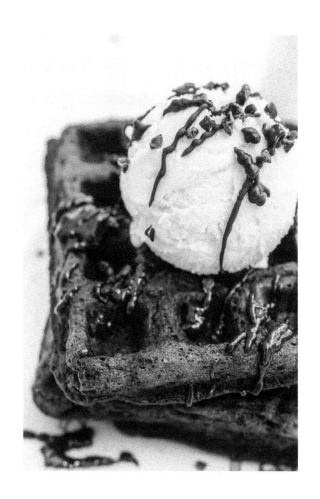

Healthy Multigrain Chia Chaffles

Preparation Time:

15 minutes

Cooking Time:

20 minutes

Serving: 8

Ingredients:

- 1 3/4 cups almond
- 1 1/4 cups whole
- milk
- wheat flour
- 1/2 cup
- 1/2 cup rolled oats
- unsweetened
- 1/4 cup flax seed
- applesauce
- meal
- 1 egg
- 4 tsp baking powder
- 2 tsp chia seeds
- 2 tsp white sugar
- 1 tsp vanilla extract
- 1/4 tsp salt

Directions:

1. Preheat a Chaffle iron shower within with cooking splash.
2. Whisk almond milk, fruit purée, egg, chia seeds, and vanilla concentrate

together in a bowl; let sit until chia seeds begin to thicken the blend, around 2 minutes.

3. Whisk flour, oats, flaxseed supper, preparing powder, sugar, and salt into almond milk blend until the batter is smooth.

4. Scoop 1/2 cup batter into the preheated Chaffle iron and cook until fresh and brilliant, around 5 minutes for each Chaffle.

5. Rehash with the rest of the batter.

Rich Yogurt Chaffles

Preparation Time:

10 minutes

Cooking Time:

20 minutes

Serving: 4

Ingredients:

- 3 eggs
- 2 tsp baking powder
- 1 1/2 cups vanilla
- 1 tsp baking soda
- fat-free yogurt
- 1/2 tsp kosher salt
- 1 1/4 cups all-
- 1/2 cup shortening
- purpose flour

Directions:

1. Preheat Chaffle iron.
2. Beat eggs in an enormous blending bowl, at that point include yogurt, flour, heating powder, preparing pop, legitimate salt, and shortening, blending until smooth.
3. Pour batter onto the hot Chaffle iron.
4. Cook until never again steaming, around 5 minutes.

Keto Chaffle Taco Shells

Preparation Time:

5 minutes

Cooking Time:

20 minutes

Servings: 5 Taco Shells

Ingredients:

- 1 tsp almond flour
- 1 cup taco blend cheese
- 2 eggs
- 1/4 tsp taco seasoning

Directions:

1. In a bowl blend almond flour, taco mix cheddar, eggs, and taco flavoring.
2. I think that it's most straightforward to blend everything utilizing a fork.
3. Include 1.5 tsp of taco chaffle hitter to the Chaffle creator at once.
4. Cook chaffle batter in the Chaffle creator for 4 minutes.
5. Remove the taco chaffle shell from the Chaffle creator and wrap over the side of a bowl. Utilized the pie container since it was what I had close by however pretty much any bowl will work.
6. Keep making chaffle taco dishes until you are out of the batter.

7. At that point fill your taco shells with taco meat, your preferred ingredients and enjoy!

Grain-Free, Low Carb Keto Chaffles

Preparation Time:

5 minutes

Cooking Time:

15 minutes

Serving: 2

Ingredients:

- 1 tsp of almond
- 1 shake of cinnamon
- flour
- 1 tsp baking powder
- 1 egg
- 1 cup mozzarella
- 1 tsp vanilla
- cheese

Directions:

1. In a bowl, combine, egg and vanilla concentrate.
2. Blend in preparing powder, almond flour, and cinnamon.
3. Finally, include the mozzarella cheddar and coat it equitably with the blend.
4. Shower your Chaffle producer with oil and let it heat up to its most noteworthy setting.

5. Cook the Chaffle, minding it at regular intervals until it gets crunchy and brilliant.
6. Making it a muddled procedure. I recommend putting down a silpat tangle for simple cleanup.
7. Take it out cautiously, and top it with spread, and your preferred low-carb syrup.

Keto Taco Chaffle

Preparation Time:

10 minutes

Cooking Time:

8 minutes

Serving: 4

Ingredients

- Chaffle:
- ¼- tsp salt
- ½- cup cheese
- ½ tsp smoked
- egg
- paprika
- ¼- tsp Italian
- ¼- cup chili powder
- seasoning
- 1/4 cup ground
- tsp chili powder
- cumin
- tsp ground cumin
- tsp garlic powder
- ½- tsp garlic
- tsp cocoa powder
- powder
- tsp onion powder
- ½- tsp cocoa
- tsp salt
- powder

- tsp smoked
- ¼- tsp onion
- Paprika
- powder

Directions:

1. Cook your floor meat or ground turkey first.
2. Include all of the taco meat seasonings. The cocoa powder is discretionary yet it clearly improves the forms of the various seasonings!
3. While you're making the taco meat, start making the keto chaffles.
4. Spot a huge part of the chaffle blend into the smaller than traditional Chaffle author and cook dinner it for around 3 to 4minutes.
5. Rehash and cook the second one 50% of the blend to make the second chaffle.
6. Add the nice and cozy taco meat to your taco chaffle. Top it with lettuce, tomatoes, cheddar, and serve warm

Keto Cornbread Chaffle Recipe

Preparation Time:

10 minutes

Cooking Time:

8 minutes

Serving: 3

Ingredients

- 1 egg
- 1 tsp Frank's Red
- 1/2 cup cheddar
- hot sauce
- cheese
- 1/4 tsp corn extract
- 5 slices jalapeno
- pinch salt

Directions:

1. Preheat the more diminutive than everyday Chaffle maker
2. In a bit bowl, whip the egg.
3. Combine the rest of the ingredients and mix it till it is all-round joined.
4. Include a tsp of shredded cheddar to the Chaffle producer for 30 seconds in advance than which comprise the order.
5. This will make a first-rate and smooth outside that is truly extraordinary

6. Add a big part of the combo to the preheated Chaffle producer.
7. Make it for at least three to 4minutes. The longer you make supper it the more energizing it receives.
8. Serve heat and respect it

Keto Chaffle Stuffing Recipe

Preparation Time:

10 minutes

Cooking Time:

35 minutes

Serving: 4

Ingredients:

- Basic Chaffle:
- 1/4 tsp salt
- 1/2 cup cheese,
- 1/4 tsp pepper
- mozzarella
- Stuffing:
- 2 eggs
- 1 small onion
- 1/4 tsp garlic
- 2 celery stalks
- powder
- 4 oz mushrooms
- 1/2 tsp onion
- 4 tbs butter
- powder
- 3 eggs
- 1/2 tsp dried
- poultry seasoning

Directions:

1. To begin with, make your chaffles. Preheat the smaller than normal Chaffle iron.
2. Preheat the stove to 350F
3. In a medium-size bowl, join the chaffle ingredients.
4. Pour a 1/4 of the blend into a smaller than expected Chaffle producer and cook each chaffle for around 4 minutes each.
5. In a little griddle, saute the onion, celery, and mushrooms until they are delicate.
6. In a different bowl, destroy the chaffles into little pieces, include the sauteed veggies and 3 eggs.
7. Blend until the ingredients are completely joined.
8. Add the stuffing blend to a little goulash dish and prepare it at 350 degrees for around 30 to 40 minutes.
9. Serve warm and enjoy

Chicken Zinger Chaffle

Preparation Time:

15 minutes

Cooking Time:

15 minutes

Servings: 2

Ingredients:

- 1 chicken breast, cut into 2 pieces
- 1/2 cup coconut flour
- 1/4 cup finely grated Parmesan
- 1 tsp. paprika
- 1/2 tsp. garlic powder
- 1/2 tsp. onion powder
- 1 tsp. salt& pepper
- 1 egg beaten
- Avocado oil for frying
- Lettuce leaves
- BBQ sauce
- Chaffle Ingredients
- 4 oz. cheese
- 2 whole eggs
- 2 oz. almond flour
- 1/4 cup almond flour
- 1 tsp baking powder

Directions:

1. Mix together chaffle ingredients in a bowl.

2. Pour the chaffle batter in preheated greased square chaffle maker.
3. Cook chaffles for about 2-3 minutes until cooked through.
4. Make 4 square chaffles from this batter.
5. Meanwhile mix together coconut flour, parmesan, paprika, garlic powder, onion powder salt and pepper in a bowl.
6. Dip chicken first in coconut flour mixture then in beaten egg.
7. Heat avocado oil in a skillet and cook chicken from both sides. until lightly brown and cooked
8. Set chicken zinger between two chaffles with lettuce and BBQ sauce.
9. Enjoy!

Chaffle & Chicken Lunch Plate

Preparation Time:

5 minutes

Cooking Time:

15 minutes

Servings: 1

Ingredients:

- 1 large egg
- 1/2 cup jack cheese, shredded
- 1 pinch salt

- For Serving
- 1 chicken leg
- salt
- pepper
- 1 tsp. garlic, minced
- 1 egg
- 1 tsp avocado oil

Directions:

1. Heat your square waffle maker and grease with cooking spray.
2. Pour Chaffle batter intothe skillet and cook for about 2-3 minutes.
3. Meanwhile,heat oil in a pan, over medium heat.
4. Once the oil is hot, add chicken thigh and garlicthen, cook for about 4-5 minutes. Flip and cook for another 3-4 minutes.
5. Season with salt and pepper and give them a good mix.
6. Transfer cooked thigh to plate.
7. Fry the egg in the same pan for about 1-2 minutes according to your choice.
8. Once chaffles are cooked, serve with fried egg and chicken thigh.
9. Enjoy!

Pork Chaffle Sandwich

Preparation Time:

5 minutes

Cooking Time:

15 minutes

Servings: 2

Ingredients:

- 1/2 cup mozzarella, shredded
- 1 egg
- I pinch garlic powder
- Pork Patty
- 1/2 cup pork, minced
- 1 tbsp. green onion, diced
- 1/2 tsp Italian seasoning
- Lettuce leaves

Directions:

1. Preheat the square waffle maker and grease with
2. Mix together egg, cheese and garlic powder in a small mixing bowl.
3. Pour batter in a preheated waffle maker and close the lid.
4. Make 2 chaffles from thisbatter.
5. Cook chaffles for about 2-3 minutes until cooked through.
6. Meanwhile, mix together pork patty ingredients in a bowl and make 1 large patty.

7. Grill pork patty in a preheated grill for about 3-4 minutes per side until cooked through.
8. Arrange pork patty between two chaffles with lettuce leaves. Cut sandwich to make a triangular sandwich.
9. Enjoy!

Crunchy Fish And Chaffle Bites

Preparation Time:

15 minutes

Cooking Time:

15 minutes

Servings: 4

Ingredients:

- 1 lb. cod fillets, sliced into 4 slice
- 1 tsp. sea salt
- 1 tsp. garlic powder
- 1 egg, whisked
- 1 cup almond flour
- 2 tbsp. avocado oil
- Chaffle Ingredients
- 2 eggs
- 1/2 cup cheddar cheese
- 2 tbsps. almond flour
- ½ tsp. Italian seasoning

Directions:

1. Mix together chaffle ingredients in a bowl and make 4 square
2. Put the chaffles in a preheated chaffle maker.
3. Mix together the salt, pepper, and garlic powder in a mixing bowl. Toss the cod cubes in this mixture and let sit for 10 minutes.

4. Then dip each cod slice into the egg mixture and then into the almond flour.
5. Heat oil in skillet and fish cubes for about 2-3 minutes, until cooked and browned
6. Serve on chaffles and enjoy!

Double Chicken Chaffles

Preparation Time:

5 minutes

Cooking Time:

5 minutes

Servings: 2

Ingredients:

- 1/2 Cup Boil Shredded Chicken
- 1/4 Cup Cheddar Cheese
- 1/8 Cup Parmesan Cheese
- 1 Egg
- 1 Tsp. Italian Seasoning
- 1/8 Tsp. Garlic Powder
- 1 Tsp. Cream Cheese

Directions:

1. Preheat the Belgian waffle maker.
2. Mix together in chaffle ingredients in a bowl and mix together.
3. Sprinkle 1 tbsp. of cheese in a waffle maker and pour in chaffle batter.
4. Pour 1 tbsp. of cheese over batter and close the lid.
5. Cook chaffles for about 4 to 5 minutes.

6. Serve with a chicken zinger and enjoy the double chicken flavor.

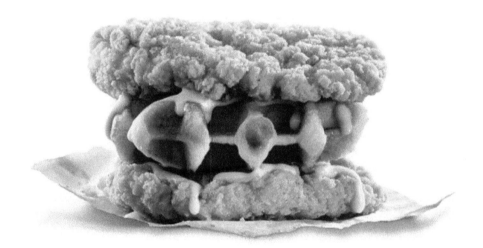

Chicken Bites With Chaffles

Preparation Time:

5 minutes

Cooking Time:

10 minutes

Servings: 2

Ingredients:

- 1 chicken breastscut into 2 x2 inch chunks
- 1 egg, whisked
- 1/4 cup almond flour
- 2 tbsps. onion powder
- 2 tbsps. garlic powder
- 1 tsp. dried oregano
- 1 tsp. paprika powder
- 1 tsp. salt
- 1/2 tsp. black pepper
- 2 tbsps. avocado oil

Directions:

1. Add all the dry ingredients together into a large bowl. Mix well.
2. Place the eggs into a separate bowl.
3. Dip each chicken piece into the egg and then into the dry ingredients.
4. Heat oil in 10-inch skillet, add oil.
5. Once avocado oil is hot, place the coated chicken nuggets onto a skillet

and cook for 6-8 minutes until
cooked and golden brown.
6. Serve with chaffles and raspberries.
7. Enjoy!

Cauliflower Chaffles And Tomatoes

Preparation Time:

5 minutes

Cooking Time:

15 minutes

Servings: 2

Ingredients:

- 1/2 cup cauliflower
- 1/4 tsp. garlic powder
- 1/4 tsp. black pepper
- 1/4 tsp. Salt
- 1/2 cup shredded cheddar cheese
- 1 egg
- For Topping
- 1 lettuce leave
- 1 tomato sliced
- 4 oz. cauliflower steamed, mashed
- 1 tsp sesame seeds

Directions:

1. Add all chaffle ingredients into a blender and mix well.
2. Sprinkle 1/8 shredded cheese on the waffle maker and pour cauliflower mixture in a preheated waffle maker and sprinkle the rest of the cheese over it.
3. Cook chaffles for about 4-5 minutes until cooked

4. For serving, lay lettuce leaves over chaffle top with steamed cauliflower and tomato.
5. Drizzle sesame seeds on top.
6. Enjoy!

Chaffle With Cheese & Bacon

Preparation Time:

15 minutes

Cooking Time:

15 minutes

Servings: 2

Ingredients:

- 1 egg
- 1/2 cup cheddar cheese, shredded
- 1 tbsp. parmesan cheese
- 3/4 tsp coconut flour
- 1/4 tsp baking powder
- 1/8 tsp Italian Seasoning
- pinch of salt
- 1/4 tsp garlic powder
- For Topping
- 1 bacon sliced, cooked and chopped
- 1/2 cup mozzarella cheese, shredded
- 1/4 tsp parsley, chopped

Directions

1. Preheat oven to 400 degrees.
2. Switch on your mini waffle maker and grease with cooking spray.
3. Mix together chaffle ingredients in a mixing bowl until combined.
4. Spoon half of the batter in the center of the waffle maker and close the lid.

Cook chaffles for about 3-4 minutes until cooked.

5. Carefully remove chaffles from the maker.
6. Arrange chaffles in a greased baking tray.
7. Top with mozzarella cheese, chopped bacon and parsley.
8. And bake in the oven for 4 -5 minutes.
9. Once the cheese is melted, remove from the oven.
10.   Serve and enjoy!

Chaffle Mini Sandwich

Preparation Time:

5 minutes

Cooking Time:

10 minutes

Servings: 2

Ingredients:

- 1 large egg
- 1/8 cup almond flour
- 1/2 tsp. garlic powder
- 3/4 tsp. baking powder
- 1/2 cup shredded cheese
- Sandwich Filling
- 2 slices deli ham
- 2 slices tomatoes
- 1 slice cheddar cheese

Directions:

1. Grease your square waffle maker and preheat it on medium heat.
2. Mix together chaffle ingredients in a mixing bowl until well combined.
3. Pour batter intoa square waffle and make two chaffles.
4. Once chaffles are cooked, remove from the maker.
5. For a sandwich,arrange deli ham, tomato slice and cheddar cheese between two chaffles.

6. Cut sandwich from the center.
7. Serve and enjoy!

Chaffles With Topping

Preparation Time:

5 minutes

Cooking Time:

10 minutes

Servings: 3

Ingredients:

- 1 large egg
- 1 tbsp. almond flour
- 1 tbsp. full-fat Greek yogurt
- 1/8 tsp baking powder
- 1/4 cup shredded Swiss cheese
- Topping
- 4oz. grill prawns
- 4 oz. steamed cauliflower mash
- 1/2 zucchini sliced
- 3 lettuce leaves
- 1 tomato, sliced
- 1 tbsp. flax seeds

Directions

1. Make 3 chaffles with the given chaffles ingredients.
2. For serving, arrange lettuce leaves on each chaffle.
3. Top with zucchini slice, grill prawns, cauliflower mash and a tomato slice.
4. Drizzle flax seeds on top.
5. Serve and enjoy!

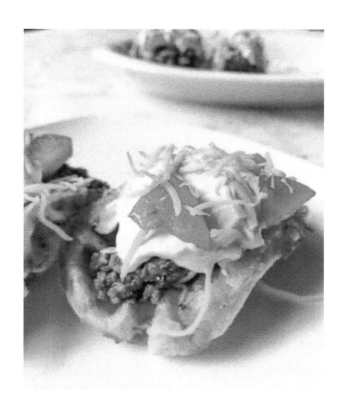